An
Issue
of
Blood

Rose Fancy

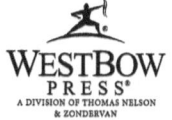

WESTBOW
PRESS®
A DIVISION OF THOMAS NELSON
& ZONDERVAN

WestBow Press books may be ordered through booksellers or by contacting:

WestBow Press
A Division of Thomas Nelson & Zondervan
1663 Liberty Drive
Bloomington, IN 47403
www.westbowpress.com
1 (866) 928-1240

ISBN: 978-1-5127-5849-8 (sc)
ISBN: 978-1-5127-5850-4 (e)

Library of Congress Control Number: 2016916196

Print information available on the last page.

WestBow Press rev. date: 10/27/2016

To Mom, Dad and my daughter,
Kitty and Chunney

Contents

Foreword

As a non-medically trained individual, I have always appreciated the depth of knowledge and commitment of many in the medical community who take their oaths seriously, especially those like my current primary care doctor. However, many individuals who have been patients have also contributed to some of the greatest breakthroughs in medicine and nutrition. Their drive to find answers to questions that sometimes the "traditional" or even "alternative" medical communities could not answer or could not answer adequately have made pioneers of many suffering patients. The author of *An Issue of Blood* is that type of pioneering patient. This is the story of how she beat endometriosis naturally and a challenge to those in the medical and nutrition arenas and to the public to test and implement her methods and plan to conqueror endometriosis and other illnesses.

Rose Fancy is proof positive that her plan works. She has been totally free of any symptoms of endometriosis for well over fifteen years. Some may be skeptical or even have some legitimate questions about what she purports. Consequently, readers are encouraged, as usual, to check with their physician before making any drastic changes to their diet. If you are cleared or simply in dire need of a solution, as was Fancy, you should still seek the "great physician" for wisdom and direction. Then make incremental adjustments or changes to your diet.

It usually takes a level of faith and courage to do something different or out of the box. That is the way to progress. So much of what is the norm today, from aviation travels to mobile phones to even laser and robotic surgeries, was once considered unthinkable or irrational. Many long-held beliefs in medicine and nutrition have changed as a result of new research studies, sometimes conducted by unlikely visionaries or theorists. Therefore, as you read the material in *An Issue of Blood*, open your heart and mind to something new or to a concept that may be the beginning of something powerful that could help thousands of suffering patients, possibly including yourself or someone you know now or in the future.

"Beloved, I wish above all things that thou mayest prosper and be in health, even as thy soul prospereth" (3 John 2 [KJV]).

A fellow sojourner on the healing pathway,
Antoinette "Toni" Mack

Preface

This book is a result of a promise I made to God that, if he revealed what was causing my illness, I would tell others. *An Issue of Blood* highlights my journey from finding out what was making me ill to what I did to overcome the illness. I was diagnosed with endometriosis, and my story seemed so similar to the woman told of in the Bible who had an issue of blood. The nutrition fact that was revealed to me during this journey is also summarized in my own theory on nutrition. I have communicated this theory to other people who have used it to overcome their illnesses.

Part I
Fancy's Story

1

Endometriosis: Naming The Pain

And a certain woman, which had an issue of blood twelve years.
—Mark 5:25

And a woman having an issue of blood twelve years, which had spent all her living upon physicians, neither could be healed of any, Came behind him, and touched the border of his garment: and immediately her issue of blood stanched.
—Luke 8:43–44

I had a happy childhood. My cat, Kitty, would come through the top-open portion of the window every Saturday morning and sleep at my feet. During the week, the family woke up early and gave Kitty something to eat. On Saturdays, we were allowed to sleep in. So Kitty would climb in through the open window to see what had happened with his breakfast. He was not our cat; he belonged to the neighborhood. He would walk from yard to yard to look for food and companionship. He visited our home daily for a period of time. Then he disappeared, only to return in two weeks.

I loved Kitty and always lifted him up like a baby. He would watch television in my lap and purr as I stroked his brown and white fur. He was my friend and sat at my feet at the dinner table. I would drop food onto the concrete floor for him. I noticed that he would eat any meat I dropped but would leave the vegetables. I would ask Daddy why Kitty ate the meat and not the vegetables. He said that cats ate meat. I noticed that Chunney, my dog, ate lots of meat also. I also observed that sometimes Kitty and Chunney ate a small amount of grass from the garden. I asked Daddy why they did that. He said they were eating the grass as medicine.

Kitty was my friend. When I did not like what was on the dinner plate, I would drop it, and he would eat it up. I learned a lot from Kitty. I watched him sit still for hours, looking. I asked Mom why he did that. She said he was looking for a lizard, and he had to be quiet and sit still so that the lizard did not know he was there. I would lie down still beside him and watch for a lizard too.

I had to sit still after dinner. If did not sit still, I would be sick. Every evening after dinner, I had to take some antacid and sit still for an hour to settle my stomach. One day, I had some pac choi and was sick. I didn't like to eat too many vegetables.

***

When the teenage years rolled by and puberty started, I experienced the usual monthly pain. I took painkillers, and I was fine. During puberty, I was sick each time I had my monthly cycle. The pain at the start of the cycle indicated the trauma that was to come. It started with diarrhea and then severe pain on the first day or two of the cycle. I had to take a painkiller to stop the pain. I also was sick after some meals, especially dinner, during my cycle. I guessed every woman had to go through this pain.

My friend Judine Scope had similar pains during her menstrual cycle. We would talk about it while walking from classes. She stayed home from school to cope with the pains. I didn't stay home from school. I loved school, and I didn't want to get behind and have to catch up on for all the missed classes. So I kept painkillers in my purse each day.

As I got older, the pain seemed more severe, and it took more painkillers to get me through my monthly cycle. One of my friends, Angelica Tate, an older woman, said that she'd had pains with her monthly cycle, but after she'd had a baby, the pain had stopped.

***

My beautiful baby was born. As I watched her sleeping soundly, I thought how beautiful she was and how glad I was that she was here. I had been sick for the entire pregnancy. The delivery was especially painful.

I now hoped I would get some relief from the pain during my monthly cycle. I had felt absolutely no pain so far. This was heaven.

A year later, I had a small amount of pain during my monthly cycle but not the excruciating pains I'd had before. This was heaven. I was looking forward to the years to come.

***

Two years later, I had to go to the doctor. The pain had started again. This time, the pain was severe. Each month, the pain lasted longer. It started one day before my monthly cycle, lasted throughout the cycle, and lingered through a day after the cycle. The pains increased over three months. They began to start a week before the beginning of my monthly cycle and would continue until a week after my cycle had ended. Soon, I was engulfed in severe pain every day. Day and night, with no letting up, the pain came. When I had my cycle, I was sick. I was in bed, doubled over in pain. It was so severe that the painkillers that had once stopped the pain for six hours only lasted an hour. I needed the doctor to prescribe stronger medicine.

I went to a gynecologist. After all, the pains had started in connection with my monthly cycle. The examination was totally embarrassing. The doctor, Tantrum Ruben, tried to figure out what was wrong with me. He took his time. He sent me to take many tests. After one test, I felt okay and did not go back to Dr. Ruben.

I can manage this pain, I told myself. *I am not a wimp.*

But when the prescription tablets were finished and the pain came back, I made another appointment to see the doctor.

Dr. Ruben and I discussed the results of the first batch of tests I had undergone. He gave me some more prescription tablets and sent me to take another batch of tests. I went and took the tests. And as before, I felt a little better and did not go back to the doctor.

When the tablets were finished and I could no longer bear the pain, I rushed back to the doctor. The final test was a laparoscopy; the doctor cut me and used an instrument to see what was inside my abdomen. He drew a diagram of the patterns of the lesion.

After a full year of observations, tests, and my not turning up for appointments, Dr. Ruben told me the pain was caused by endometriosis. He gave me a pamphlet to read about the disease and the correct pills to ease the pain. The good news was that I now knew what was wrong with me. The bad news was that there was no cure.

I was glad that I finally was able to find out what my medical problem was. I had had this terrible pain for so many years, and now I was able to unmask it. I was happy to finally put a name to the pain. I knew that once I could identify the condition, I could set about finding a solution.

2

A Choice: Trying Surgery

According to the medical books, endometriosis is a condition where the lining of the uterus appears on other parts of the body. When a woman has her monthly cycle, other parts of her body bleed. This causes severe pains.

The prescription tablets provided temporary relief, and I went back to the doctor every three months for more. The pains occurred more frequently—to the point I was in severe pain every day—so I had to take the pills every day. At first I took them every four hours. But soon, I had to take them every three hours to get rid of the pain.

One holiday, I was out of medication. I was in so much pain that I went to the doctor's office, only to find it closed. I frantically called various doctors' offices to see if anyone was open. I needed a prescription to make it through the intense pain I was experiencing. I felt so sick that I wound up going to the emergency room.

I decided that enough was enough. I had to try something else to overcome the pain. I had a discussion with my doctor, and he suggested an operation to fix the lesions. He warned that this operation might or might not work. For some people, the pain disappeared, and for others, it reappeared; it worked for some patients but not for everyone. I scheduled the operation, as I could not take another day of pain.

It was set for two months later. During the months leading up to the procedure, the pain was particularly awful. That was when a coworker, Mogi Olli, told me of a Dr. Black, who practiced holistic medicine. She said I should get a second opinion. Dr. Black worked as a physician at the hospital during the day and practiced holistic medicine during the evenings and weekends. As usual, I waited until I was in severe pain to set up the appointment.

I was bent over in pain as I crawled into Dr. Black's office. He took a detailed history of my condition. He hooked me up to a machine that gave a tape of the results. From this tape, Dr. Black told me that I had been born with a weak liver and that I needed to go on a vegetarian diet to overcome the pain. I thanked him and said to myself, *Are you serious?* I was quite slim. At five foot eight, I weighed just 110 pounds. If I ate a vegetarian diet, I reasoned, I would lose even more weight. And I couldn't afford to do that.

I now had a choice. I could either have the operation, or I could try a vegetarian diet. The operation was expensive. But if I had it, I might get rid of the pain forever. It could fix the pain once and for all. That would be it—I wouldn't have any more problems for the rest of my life. On the other hand, while the vegetarian diet option was tempting, I didn't even know if it could possibly work. Plus, my concerns about my slimness and my desire not to lose more weight factored in. I decided to have the operation.

***

For six months after the operation, I was on steroids to prevent me from having a monthly cycle. I felt like a million bucks. I was finally free from the pain that had plagued me for such a long time. I was able to run and exercise. I was having the time of my life. I was very thankful to my doctor. I had to take six months of medication, and that would be it. I was free of pain.

After the operation, I left home, moved from the small island I had been living on to the mainland, and settled into a new job and new apartment. Life was good. The job I'd found was temporary. It didn't provide benefits such as health insurance. But I was in need of a job, so I took it. I was on my own for the first time. I had enough strength to work and do my housework unaided. Previously, when I'd been living on the small island, I'd had a helper or a maid who came in each day to clean and cook during the week. When I came home from work, I would eat and go to sleep. That was how I had coped with the severe pain.

The mainland was a new place. I started to enjoy the food, visiting a different restaurant every weekend.

3

The Pain Returns: A New Diagnosis?

After a year on the job I felt a small pain in my side, but I ignored it. After all, it wasn't as bad as the tremendous pain I had been feeling a year and a half ago. I went on vacation for two weeks.

While on vacation I felt a slight pain and realized I could not continue to ignore the pain. I went to see a doctor. Dr. Knut said he thought that the endometriosis pain was recurring. He sent me to another doctor..

After the examinations, I was in severe pain. I went to bed bent into a coil.

The doctor informed me that I did not have endometriosis, but I had a bad case of fibroids. They were so bad that they had adhered to the walls of my uterus. He suggested I have a hysterectomy.

I did not have the money to cover such a procedure. I was a temporary employee, and so I did not have any health insurance. But how could my previous doctor, Dr. Ruben, have gotten it so wrong? Why had he told me I had endometriosis when this doctor was saying I had fibroids? Who should I believe—Dr. Ruben or this new doctor? I was confused and in severe pains and had no money to pay for further assessment *or* the hysterectomy that the doctor had suggested.

I began to regret my decision to leave the small island. There, I'd had two health insurers and had been fully covered. Here on the mainland, I was a temporary employee and did not receive any benefits. I began to wish I had stayed on the small island.

I called Nana Kit, who lived on the mainland in the north. She was a good friend and knew about my previous bouts with endometriosis. I told Nana everything. We spoke for a long time. We were both sad. We discussed the pain, the new diagnosis, and the fact that I did not have health coverage and so could not afford another operation. Talking to her was comforting and calmed me down.

After the vacation, I went to work grunting and groaning in pain. That was the only way I could cope with the pain, which was ten times worse than the pain I'd had to deal with before the operation. The pain was on the surface of my left leg, the back of my left hip, and deep in my left side.

Ms. Gorki, my supervisor. asked me what was wrong. I told her about my endometriosis, my recent doctor visit and examination, and my new diagnosis. She asked me if the doctor had given me a prescription for pain medication. In my confused state, I had forgotten to ask for a prescription, and he hadn't given me any. So you can imagine the pain I was in.

Ms. Gorki telephoned the doctor immediately and asked him to send a prescription to the nearest pharmacy. I went and picked it up.

This prescription was different from any of the medications I had taken previously. The pharmacist explained that this painkiller was a narcotic. I couldn't take it if I would be driving. If the police stopped me, I would test positive for narcotics and could be jailed. So I could not take it before driving to work. I was single and had to drive myself to work every morning.

The directions on the bottle instructed me to take the pills every six hours. Each dose, once it kicked in about three hours after I'd taken it, relieved the pain for about three hours. Then I would be in pain again. So I would take my brave self to work in severe pain, at which point I would eat and then quickly take my tablets. I would grunt and groan for three hours until the pain stopped. I sometimes tried to suck in the pain.

It was such a relief to go home from work and just lie down. The situation wasn't working. The pain was too severe. My young daughter had to do the housework.

4

A Note under the Pillow: Praying for a Miracle

I began to pray. I had been a Christian all my life, and I needed help. Most days, I would lie on the bed groaning and praying and asking God for some relief from the pain.

It was during one of my groaning sessions that my daughter, who was five years old, wrote a letter to God and asked him if he could help Mommy with her pain. She showed it to me and said, "Mommy, I am going to place this under your pillow."

The next day, when she was making up my bed, she couldn't find the note under my pillow. We searched for it. But we could not find it.

She looked and me, her eyes wide with disbelief, and said, "Mommy, we cannot find the note because God is going to answer your prayers."

She was so serious that I believed her too.

My friend Mr. Hapenten, a devout Christian, told me to pray and ask God for a miracle. I told him that there was no cure for endometriosis. He reminded me of the Bible passage that said, "And many lepers were in Israel in the time of Eliseus the prophet; and none of them was cleansed, saving Naaman the Syrian" (Luke 4:27 [KJV]). Mr. Hapenten told me to ask for a miracle. I prayed and asked God to heal not only me but also reveal to me what was causing the pain. I asked him to show me what I could do to overcome the pain, so that I could get better and help others as well.

I would go to bed at nights and take the pill and then wait for three hours it took for the pain to subside to pass. For those hours, I would pray and call on the name of the Lord. As the pain would rack my body, I would cry out, "Jesus, please help me," and, "Lord, have mercy." I would chant aloud, "Lord, please heal me." Every night I would sleep for three hours, and then the pain would return and kick me out of my sleep. The process would start over again. I would take another tablet and pray and call on the Lord's name for three hours as I again waited for the pain to subside so I could go back to sleep.

Since I did not have insurance options through my place of employment, I bought a private insurance option. It paid only a hundred dollars per visit, as well as a hundred dollars toward any medical emergency or procedure.

When I could no longer tolerate the pain, I went to the emergency room. I was surrounded by a group of doctors in training, and I felt horrible. I was referred to a gynecological specialist. When I called to make an appointment, I was told the doctor couldn't schedule me in for another three months. The pain I was dealing with at this point was tremendous, and the painkillers I had wouldn't last that long.

I asked the scheduler if I could please get an earlier appointment.

"Are you having a baby?" she asked.

"No," I said.

"Are you having a difficult pregnancy?"

"No," I told her.

"Then what is your problem?" she asked.

I tried to tell her that I was in severe pain.

"It can wait," she said.

***

A friend, Elsa Bunt, heard me moaning and asked me about my problem. I told her. She gave me the name of her gynecologist, Dr. Jane Comp, along with some good advice: "Walk until you find a doctor who is saying the same thing you are saying." That is, find a doctor who will listen to what you are saying.

About this time, I found a permanent position that offered health insurance. However, I had been without health insurance for more than a year, so the insurance company refused to cover anything deemed a "preexisting condition." In other words, my insurer would not cover treatment for endometriosis. I would have to pay the insurance premiums for a year before the health insurance would cover any costs associated with treating my endometriosis. I would have to continue to endure this pain for another year.

Dr. Jane Comp was very nice. She listened to me carefully. I explained that I had endometriosis and that I was in pains. I told her about my confusion because of the two different diagnoses I'd received—that Dr. Ruben had said I was suffering from endometriosis, while the doctor had said fibroids was the culprit.

Dr. Comp asked me what type of tests Dr. Ruben had ordered, and I listed them. In addition to telling her about the various tests I'd undergone, I told her about the laparoscopy and the diagram and diagnosis that had followed, as well as the resulting operation. I told her about the steroid series I'd taken for six months and my temporary belief I'd been cured and how the pain had returned and had grown more and more severe ever since. I told her about visiting to the doctor and the painful examinations, along with his fibroid diagnosis and recommendation that I have a hysterectomy. I told her I couldn't afford to pay for the operation, as my current health insurer considered it treatment of a preexisting condition.

She asked me what type of test the doctor had ordered before making the fibroids diagnosis, and I told her I hadn't undergone any tests. She explained that she believed I had endometriosis, as Dr Ruben had been thorough in his analysis and had conducted several tests. She wanted me to transfer my medical history to her. In the meantime, she gave me a free sample of pain medication that some pharmaceutical company had given her. She told me that stress was associated with endometriosis and that, when I was unable to work, it was okay to lie down.

I took the medication. When the free tablets were gone, I went back to Dr. Comp. Lucky for me, she had some other samples, but these pills had to be embedded in my abdomen each month. When those samples were gone, I started to fret. I did not have any money to buy the prescription I would need. The medication that had worked best was so expensive it would take my entire two weeks' temporary pay to fill the prescription for a month.

Dr. Comp prescribed a different medication. This one stopped the pain, but the side effect was a debilitating weakness. I could hardly walk. I took a great deal of effort to get out of bed.

I prayed daily for a miracle.

5

A Biblical Problem and a Dietary Solution

In fall 1998, I received a package from Nana Kit. I opened it to find a magazine and, in particular, an article on endometriosis that she had found while visiting a doctor's office on the northern part of the country. She'd purchased a copy and sent it to me. The article summarized a report on studies on the liver and made a connection between endometriosis and the liver. It recommended a vegetarian diet for persons with endometriosis. I asked myself where I had heard this before.

Then I remembered the holistic doctor I'd seen two years earlier. He'd recommended a vegetarian diet, and I hadn't listened. *Well*, I said to myself, *if I have to eat grass to get rid of this severe, debilitating pain, I am willing to do just that*. I was sick of being sick and tired of being tired. And I was sick and tired of being sick and sick and tired of being tired.

At this point, I was willing to try anything. It was about 9:00 p.m., and I marched to the supermarket. I was not willing to wait another day. I bought some lettuce. Why lettuce? Because I liked it.

I ate lettuce for dinner that day. That same night, for the first time in about seven years, I felt well enough to cook and clean the house. I could not believe it. What a miracle. Suddenly, I felt better.

I ate lettuce for breakfast, lunch, and dinner for about a month. I was too afraid to eat anything that might trigger the pain. I added carrots, and I still felt okay. I started to lose weight after a time because I was too afraid to add any other foods. I went from a size 12 to a size 6. I was not troubled as I had always been slim. The steroid I'd taken after the operation had caused me to move from a size 6 to a size 12.

Then one day, a friend who knew me from the small island visited.

When he saw me, he said, "It's okay if you go. I'll take care of your daughter."

The next day, I went to the public library and borrowed books on nutrition. I read extensively about the topic.

I started to add one vegetable each week to see how it affected me before I added it to the list of foods I could eat. I kept a log of things I could or couldn't eat. I went to work and told my friends what I was doing.

One woman pointed me to the Bible, specifically the book of Daniel, noting that Daniel was a vegetarian as well. (See Daniel 1:12).

***

The pain on the surface of my left leg was gone, and the pain in the back of my hip slowly disappeared as well. Both of these pains seemed to be related to the consumption of too much meat.

Soon, the pain deep in my side was gone also. It seemed to be related to the consumption of oily foods. So I boiled my food instead of frying it.

I always tried to stick to my new diet. However, one day I decided to eat a hamburger, as I hadn't tried on in a long time. After about an hour, the severe pain started back up. I was screaming in pain. I started eating the vegetables and fruits in my house to get rid of the pain. I found out that, if I ate boiled cabbage, the pain what stop. It was horrible, but it confirmed that I needed to eat a vegetarian diet.

I continued to eat only vegetables. To my surprise, the rashes on my hands and face (eczema) and in my hair (dermatitis) cleared up, and I no longer had indigestion after I ate. I wasn't sick any more after meals. I also began to put on weight, and my back stopped aching. I was no longer bone tired all the time.

Next, I added fruits to my diet, and then rice and potatoes as well. I ate a vegetarian diet 99 percent of the time, and all my pains were gone.

I stopped going to my doctors, including my gynecologist. I threw out my pain medication. I decide that this was it. And I felt angry at my doctors.

One day, I bumped into my Dr. Comp at the mall. It had been about five years since I'd been to her or any other doctor at this point. Dr. Comp asked me what had happened to me. I told her about my vegetarian diet and that I was feeling much better. She congratulated me and encouraged me to continue what I was doing and to let her know the results.

A friend of mine, Alicia Nash, told her doctor about my recovery— that I'd had endometriosis and had suffered terrible pains and that I had recovered by eating a vegetarian diet. He said that meant endometriosis was a gastrointestinal problem and not a gynecological problem as previously thought.

One day, I had a cold, and I went to Dr. Knut. He was happy to see me. He asked me how my recovery was going, and I told him about how eating a vegetarian diet had overcome the pains. He was very happy that I was healthy, and he encouraged me to go to the farmers market and eat the type of foods that I'd usually eaten when I was on the small island. My anger toward doctors suddenly disappeared.

One day, I was reflecting on everything I had been through, and I thought about the woman with the issue of blood in the Bible. It seems likely that she'd had endometriosis. I saw many similarities between her story and the experience I went through. I could understand why she had touched just the hem of Jesus' garment because she was so embarrassed by the disease that afflicted her and in so much pain. I could also understand why she had spent all her money on physicians to find a cure. I was honored to know that my disease was mentioned in the Bible.

6

Refinements: A Change for Life

After menopause, I was glad to be in a new phase of life. I decided to start eating meat again. This time, I ate one huge fish per day.

One day, suddenly, I couldn't walk, and I felt numb. I went to see a doctor, who was unable to find anything wrong with me. I went to Dr. Knut, and he sent me to a neurologist, Dr. Pulp.

Dr. Pulp said that I had stress and too much protein in my blood. He told me to take a week off of work and said that, if my protein level wasn't down by the time I took the next test, he would have to give me medication to reduce the level.

I left the doctor quickly. I knew what the problem was. I went back to my vegetarian diet. My protein levels on the next test results were good. My strength came back slowly, and I could walk again.

I realized that the vegetarian diet was for life. I finally accepted that I was born vegetarian.

***

I was watching television one day when I was recovering from stress and saw a film on animals in Africa. The film showed plant-eating animals and flesh-eating animals all congregating at water hole. I realized that, within the animal king, there were two ways of getting nutrition. Herbivores, like the elephants and the giraffes, ate plants, and carnivores, like dogs and cats, ate flesh. I recalled how, during my childhood, I had observed Kitty and Chunney eating small amounts of grass. I realized that carnivores ate a small amount of plants, so it seemed that herbivores should eat a small amount of meat.

I started to eat meat but only a small portion. From my research, I had also learned that humans need vitamin B12 to survive. Vitamin B12 is only obtained from animal meat. If you don't eat meat at all, you'll need to get your vitamin B12 in pill form. I started eating the equivalent of half an egg of meat per meal. That seemed to do the trick. Too much meat was not good for me.

Pondering the television show, I wondered if humans could also be classified as herbivores and carnivores. The classifications for humans are vegetarians and people who eat meat. I knew that natural vegetarians were people with endometriosis, stress, and depression. But who were the natural meat eaters?

I used the flashlight of my mind to peer into the darkness of possibilities, and I realized that people with diabetes were among those who should be eating meat. I could not identify any other diseases that fell into the "meatarian" category.

I called a friend, Lis Jack. Lis and I had always had a good relationship. We discussed this theory I was considering, trying to identify who the meatarians were? I had placed people with mental illness in the category of vegetarians, but as Lis and I discussed the topic, I realized that was incorrect. I did a quick survey of my friends with mental illness (violent behavior)(). They all had someone in their family who had diabetes.

I realized that mental illness could occur for two nutritional reasons. First, people who are born vegetarian who eat too much meat can become mentally ill. Second, people who are born meatarian and eat too much starchy food can become mentally ill. I decided to show this classification of humans on what I've dubbed "Fancy's Nutrition Spectrum," which will be explained in the next chapter.

I also became aware of the need to open windows to let in the breath of life. I had gone from opening all the windows in the house all day on the small island to leaving all my windows on the mainland closed because I now had air-conditioning. However, the lack of fresh air was making me ill. So I threw open the windows in spring, summer, and autumn. During winter, I opened at least two windows to let in the air. I started feeling better as soon as I'd opened the windows in my house again.

I realized too that sleep was very important. I needed eight to ten hours of sleep per day to feel refreshed. There was also the problem of daylight saving time. This caused my usual sleep pattern to be thrown off. I started to go to bed the same time each day. So when it was Eastern Standard Time, I slept from 8:00 p.m. to 4:30 a.m., and during daylight saving time, I slept from 9:00 p.m. to 5:30 a.m. The shift allowed me to be asleep at the same time each day.

I also noticed something peculiar. On the small island where I grew up, which was considered a developing country, people mainly planted food. Meat was expensive, and so people tended to eat a diet that was closer to a vegetarian diet than the typical diet on the mainland—the typical island diet was 80 percent plant-based and 20 percent meat-based. The common diseases I encountered while I was growing up were diabetes and mental illness.. On the mainland, which was considered a developed country, people ate much more meat; the typical diet was 60 percent meat-based and 40 percent plant-based. There, common diseases were endometriosis and depression.

Part II
Fancy's Nutrition Plan

7

Fancy's Nutrition Spectrum

Fancy's Nutrition Spectrum details my theory on nutrition. Human nutrition is very complex. Animals eat food according to their species, while humans eat food based on their diseases. Cows, horses, elephants, and giraffes eat plants. On the other hand, dogs and cats eat meat.

Carnivores (meat eaters)
Wolves
Lions
Dogs

Herbivores (plant eaters)
Cows
Horses
Elephants
Giraffes

Human beings are less easy to categorize, as people eat food according to their diseases (or they should). People with endometriosis, skin problems, indigestion, slim builds (accompanied by the inability to gain weight), indigestion, heart diseases, backaches, and some forms of mental illness (depression and stress-related issues) are born vegetarians. On the other hand, people who have diabetes and other forms of mental illness (violent behavior) are born meatarians.

Meatarians
Diabetes
Mental illness (Violent)

Vegetarians
Endometriosis
Inability to gain weight
Stress-related issues and depression
Indigestion
Backache
Skin problems
Panic attack syndrome
Mental illness (depression)

Humans must eat a combination of meats and plants to survive. The portion of an individual's diet that should be made up of either plant food or meat depends on the type of diseases that show up during his or her life. Fancy's Nutrition Spectrum shows different combinations of meat and plant food that humans can eat. It ranges from a meatarian diet at one end of the spectrum to a vegetarian diet at the other end of the spectrum. This model calculates the amount of plant and meat that a person can eat at each part of the spectrum and gives suggested eating portions.

Fancy's Nutrition Spectrum encourages meatarians to eat a small portion of vegetables and vegetarians to eat a small portion of meat. It is important for all persons to eat all types of food, but the portions differ depending on where an individual falls along the spectrum.

The right "size" diet

Just as some people are born boys and others are born girls, human's beings are born to eat a certain diet in order to be healthy. A person who wears size 16 shoes cannot wear a size 5. If he or she attempts to do so (and can manage to get a foot into the shoe), he or she will be in pain. Likewise, a person who wears size 5 shoes cannot wear a size 16. If he or she tries to do so, the shoes will fall off his or her feet. So it is with the human diet. If a natural vegetarian eats too much meat, then one or more of the diseases associated with natural vegetarians will manifest in his or her life. If a natural meatarian eats too much plant food, one or more of the diseases listed under meatarian will manifest during his or her life.

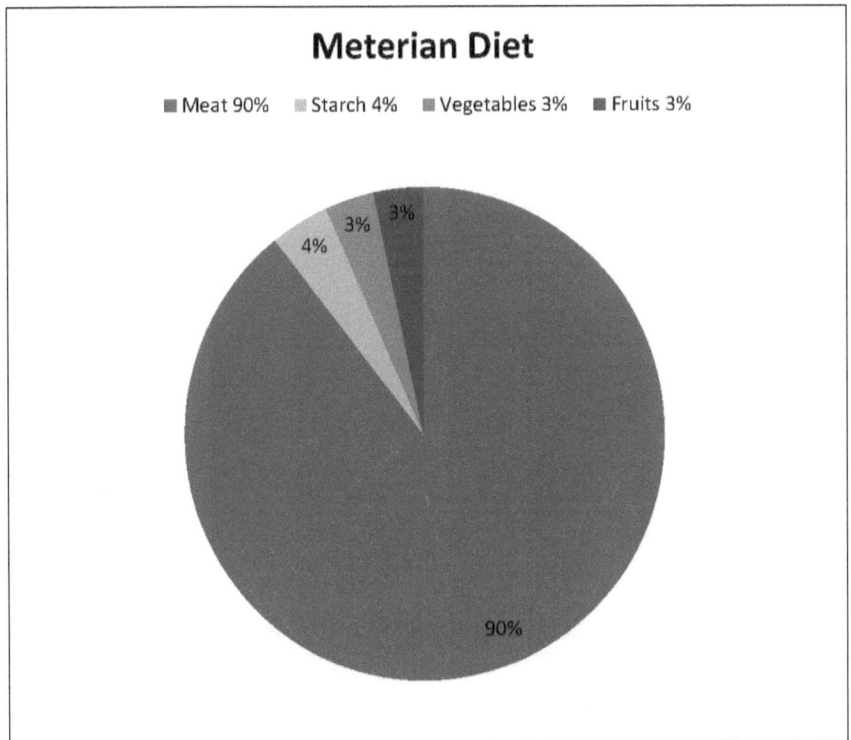

Meatarians (primarily eat meat)

At one end of Fancy's Nutrition Spectrum is the meatarian diet. People who are born meatarian should eat mainly meat. They must eat some plant food, such as vegetables, starch, and fruits to be healthy. However the portion of the plant food for the meatarian diet ranges from 10 percent to 1 percent.

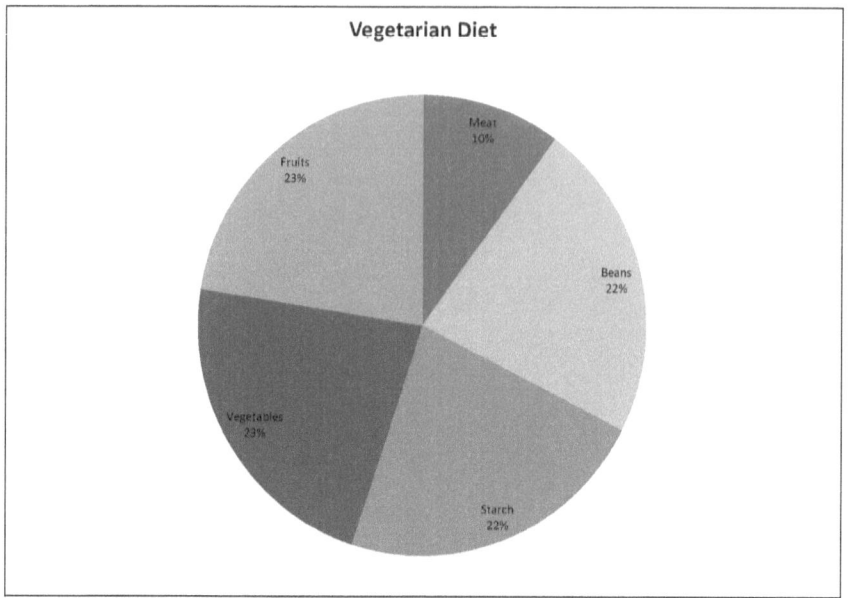

Vegetarians (primarily eat plants)

At the other end of Fancy's Nutrition Spectrum is the vegetarian diet. People who are born vegetarian should eat mainly plant food. They must eat some meat. However, the portion of meat to be eaten by vegetarians ranges from 10 percent to 1 percent.

Statistics

In statistics, the graph below is called the bell curve. This graph shows the normal pattern of human behavior. When it comes to diet, as the graph demonstrates, the majority of people eat between 89 percent meat and 11 percent plant food and 11 percent meat and 89 percent plant food and remain healthy.

However, those who fall on the ends of the spectrum—those who should eat 90 percent meat and 10 percent plant food and below (natural meatarians) and those who should eat 10 percent meat and 90 percent plant food and below (natural vegetarians)—have to careful with their diet.

If you are born a vegetarian, and you eat too much meat, you can get endometriosis, indigestion, or skin rashes and suffer from mental illness (depression), stress, or backaches. If you are born a meatarian, and you eat too much plant food, you can get diabetes and mental illness (violent behavior).

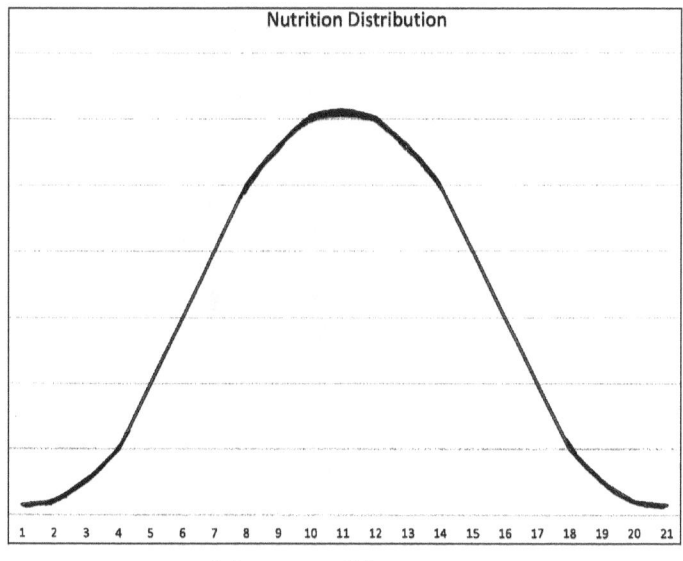

Meatarian, Vegetarian

The Normal Diet

According to the graph above, most people (that is three-quarters of the earth's population) eat a combination of foods from the normal range and remain healthy. The normal range shows all the combinations of meat and plant ranging from 89 percent meat and 11 percent plant to 11 percent meat and 89 percent plant.

Fancy's Nutrition Spectrum shows various diets that human beings can eat to be healthy. These dietary options range from being 99 percent meat-based and 1 percent plant-based to being 1 percent meat-based and 99 percent plant-based. The choice of which diet pattern to use to remain healthy depends on the disease(s) that shows up in your life. People with endometriosis, stress-related issues and mental illness (depression). should eat a vegetarian diet. People with diabetes and mental illnesses (violent behavior) should eat a meatarian diet.

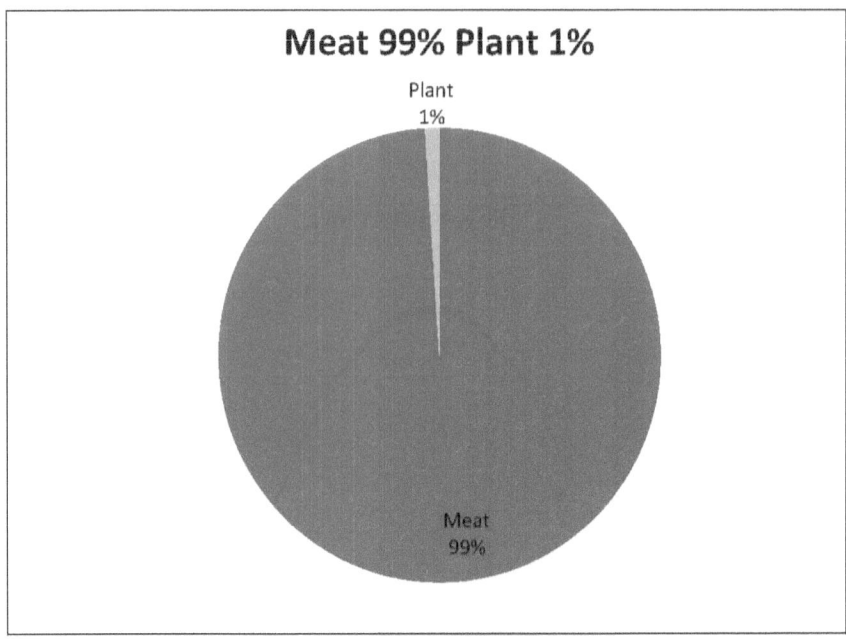

Figure: FNS1

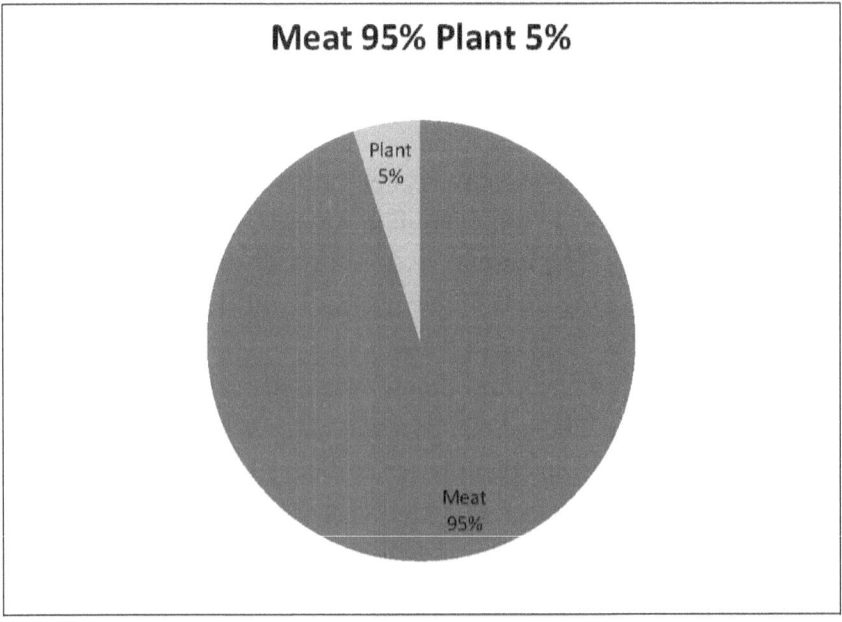

Figure: FNS2

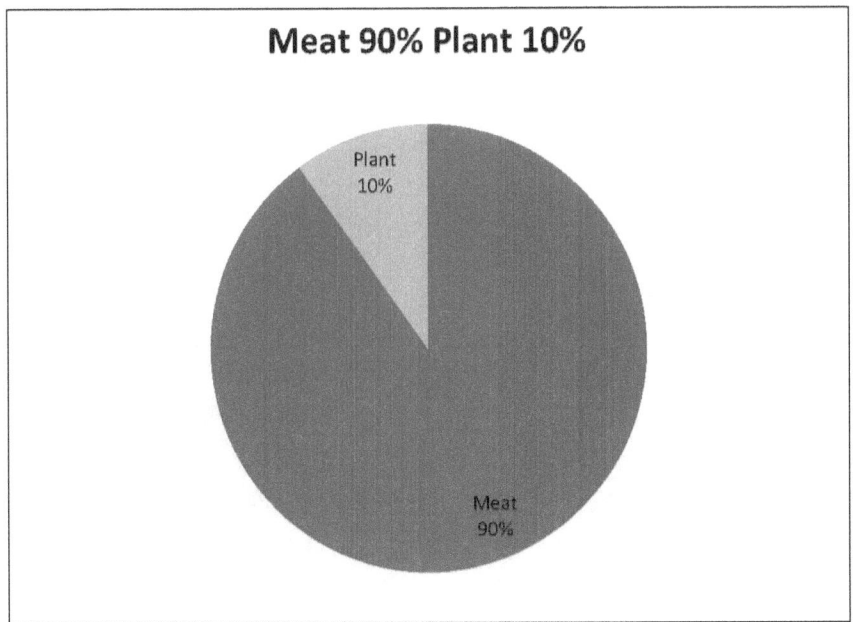

Figure: FNS3

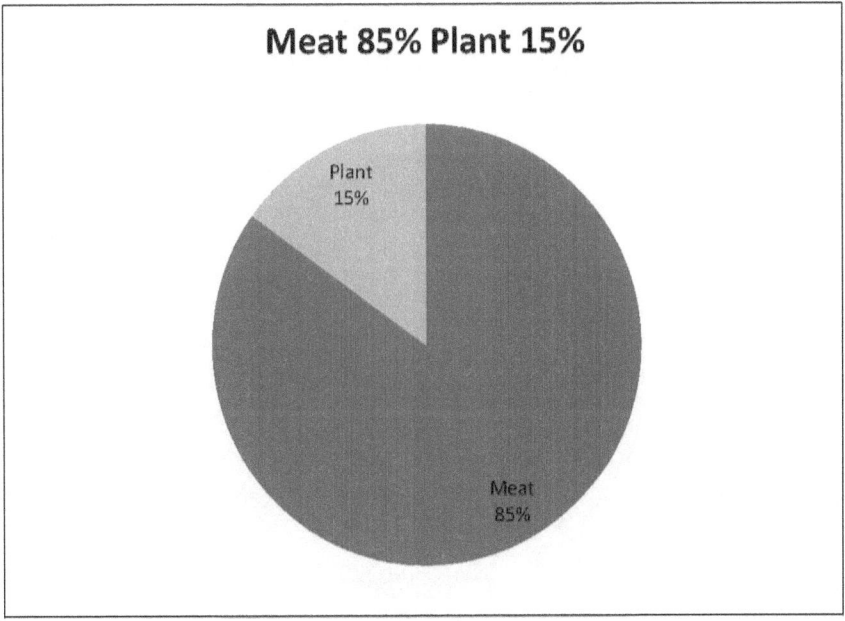

Figure: FNS4

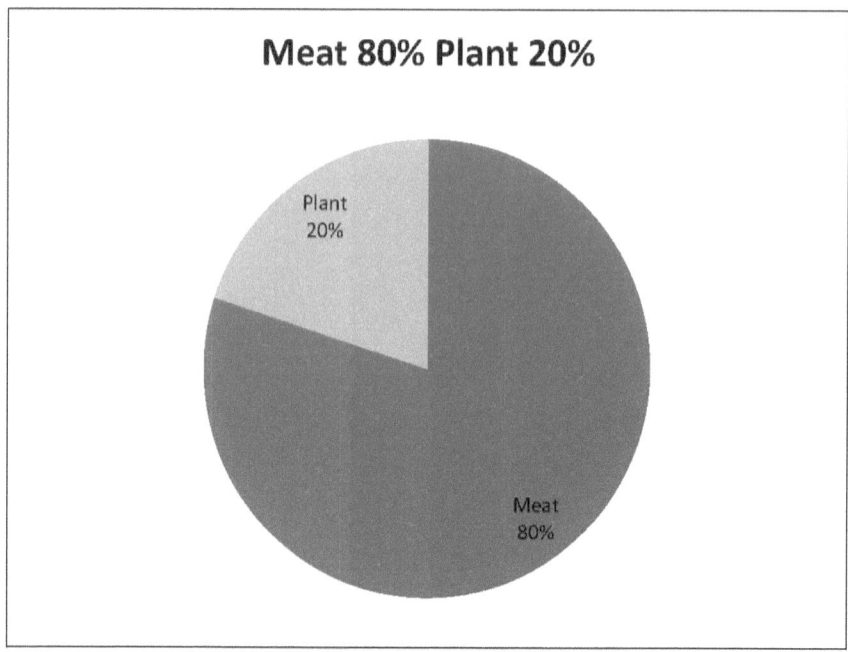

Figure: FNS5

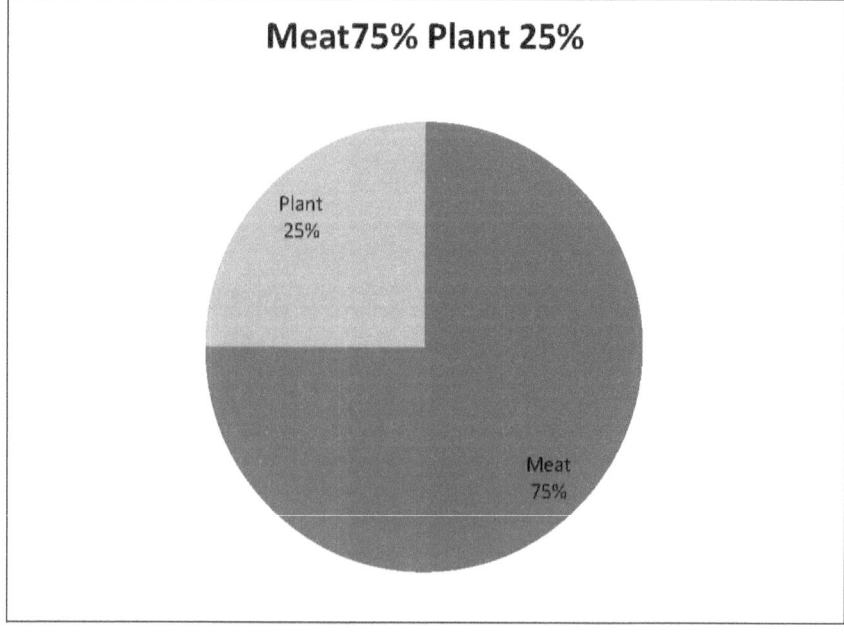

Figure: FNS6

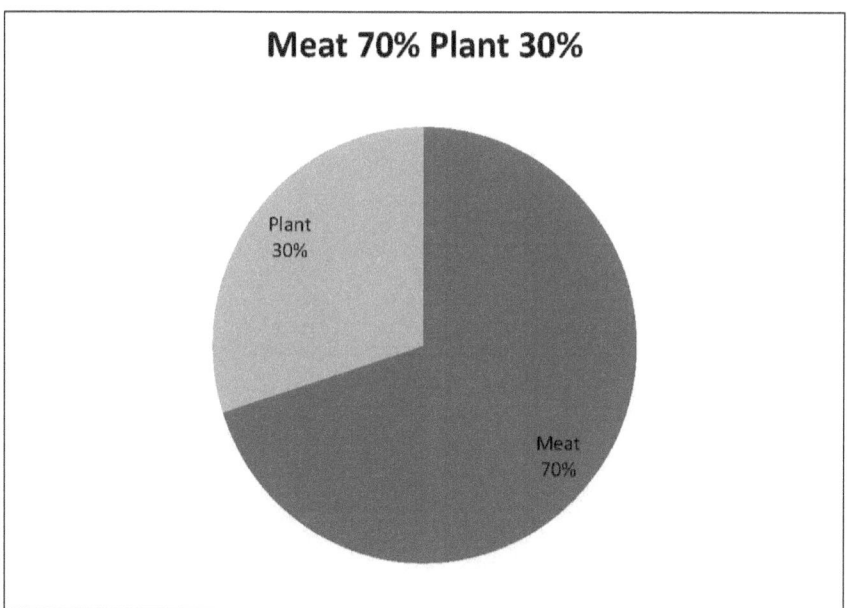

Figure: FNS7

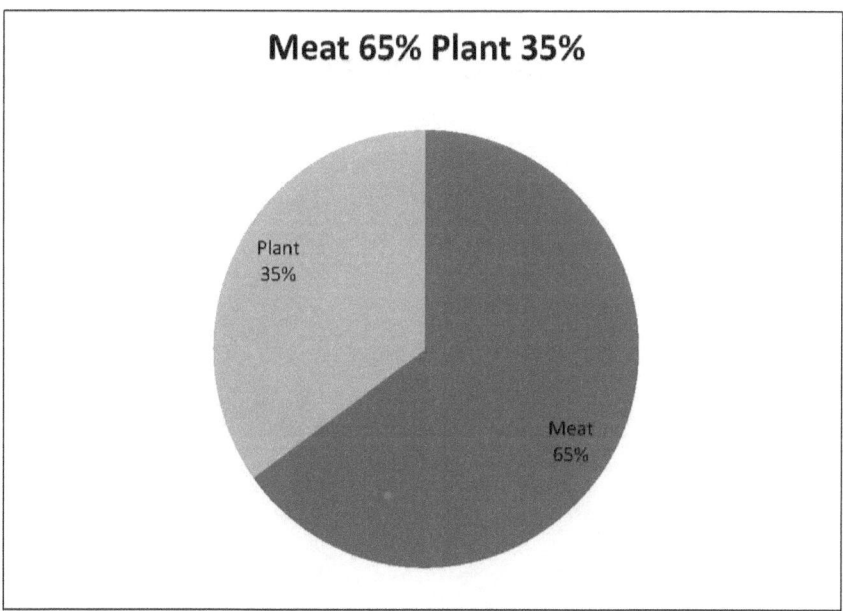

Figure: FNS8

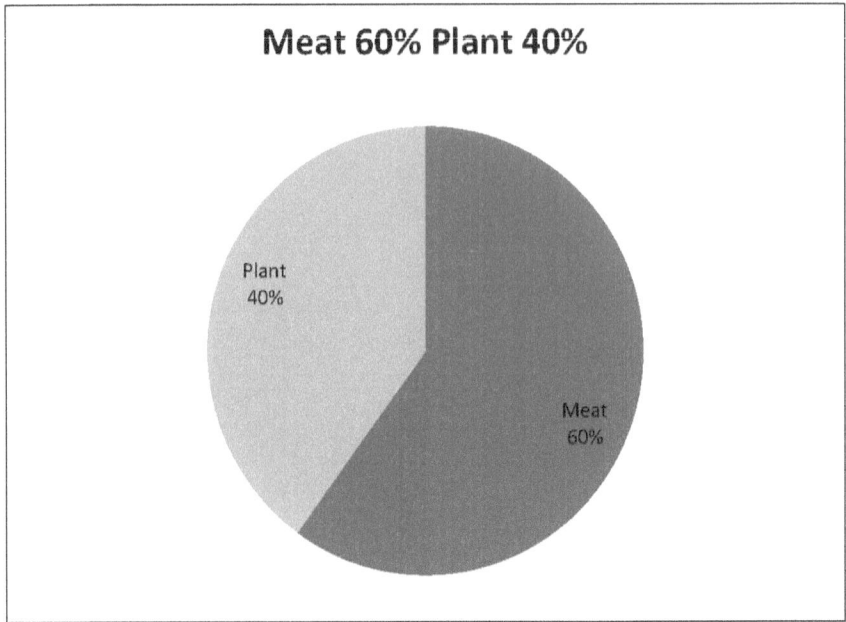

Figure: FNS9

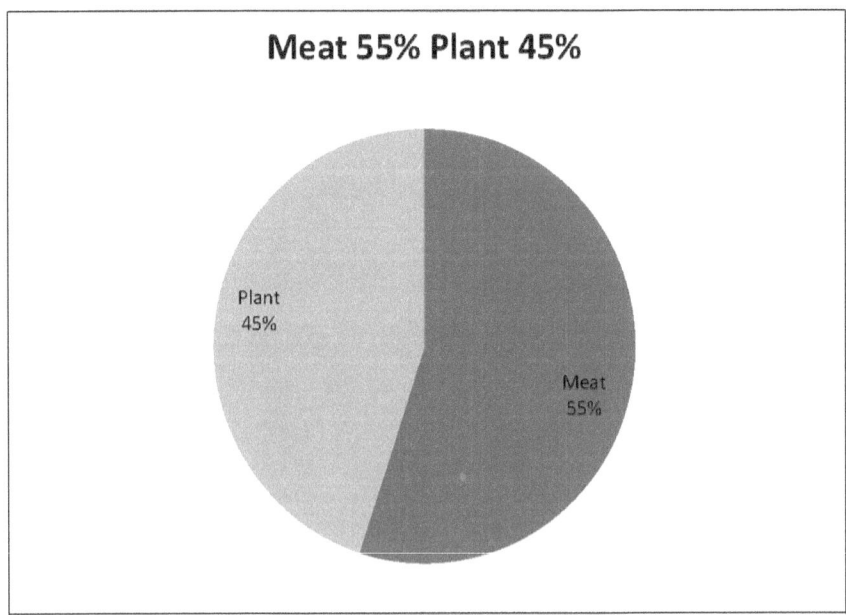

Figure: FNS10

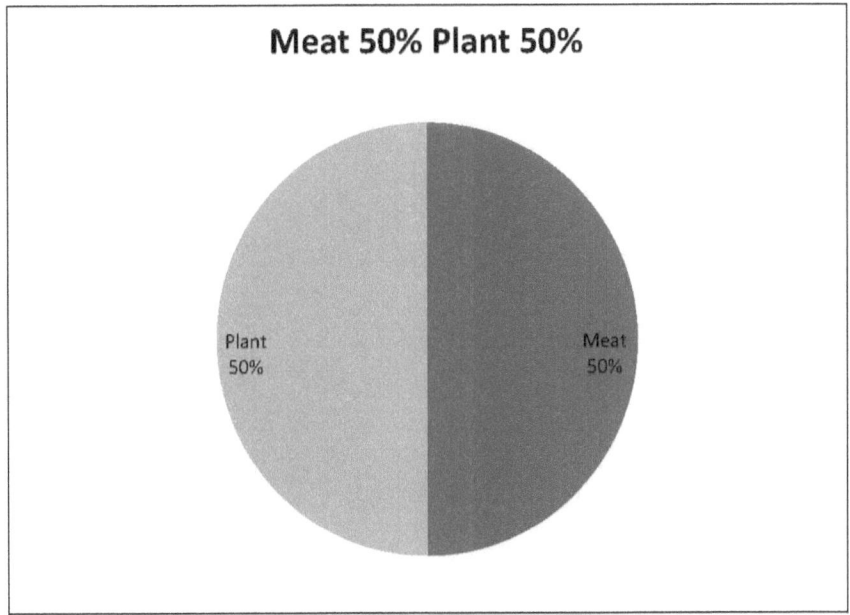

Figure: FNS11

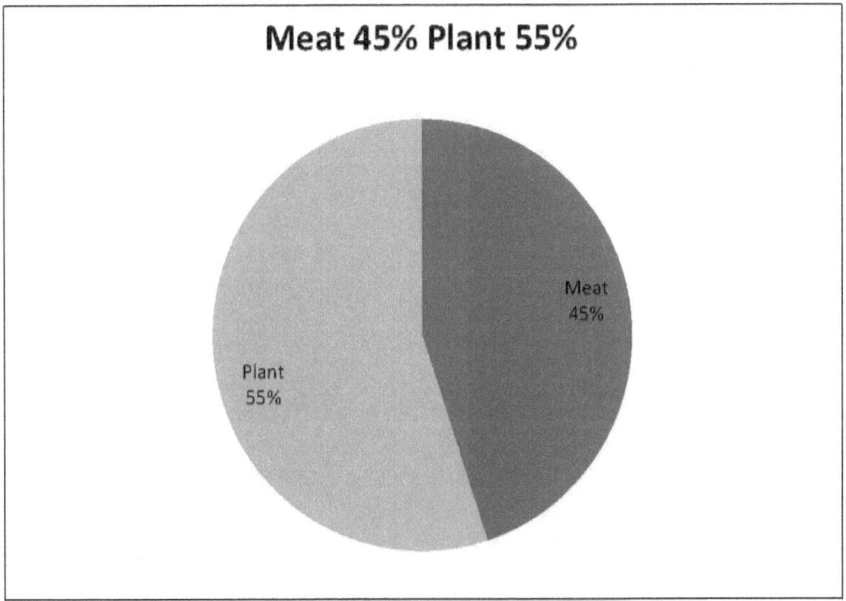

Figure : FNS12

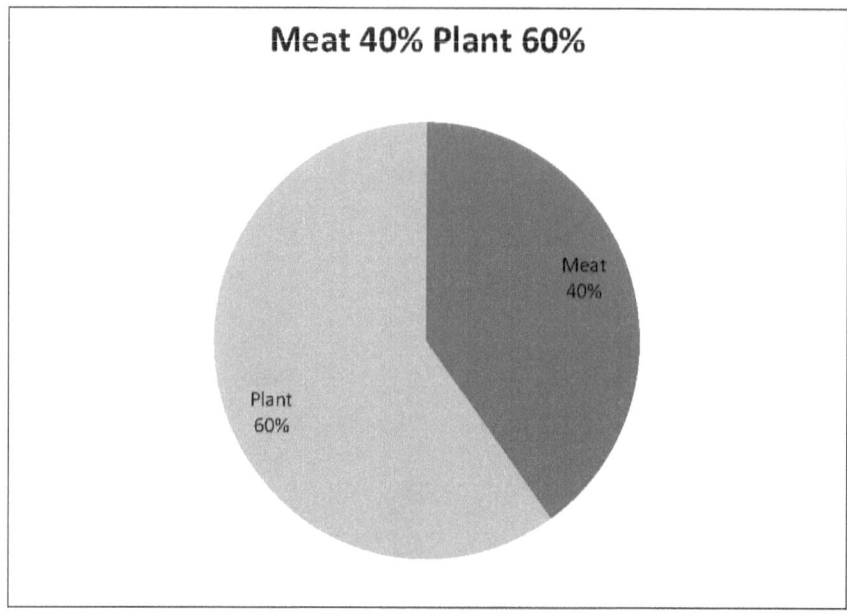

Figure: FNS13

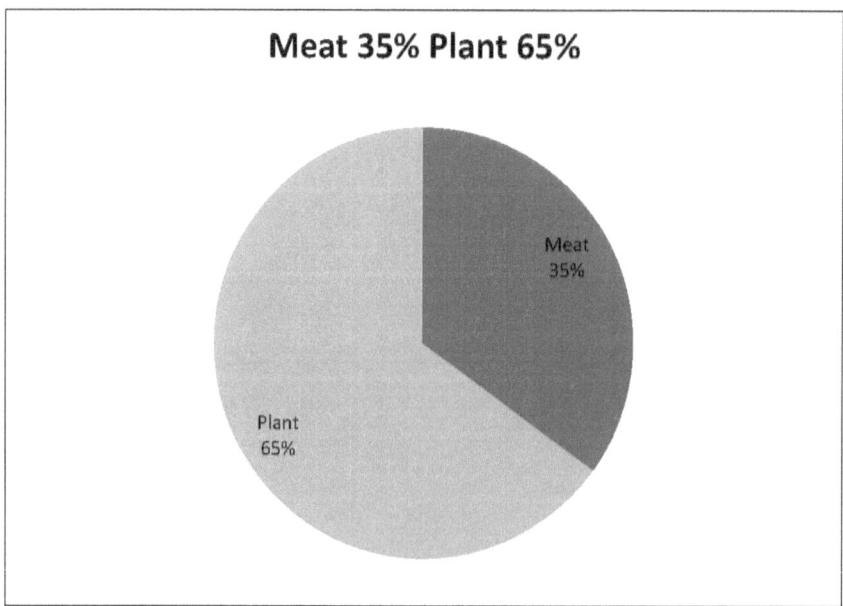

Figure: FNS14

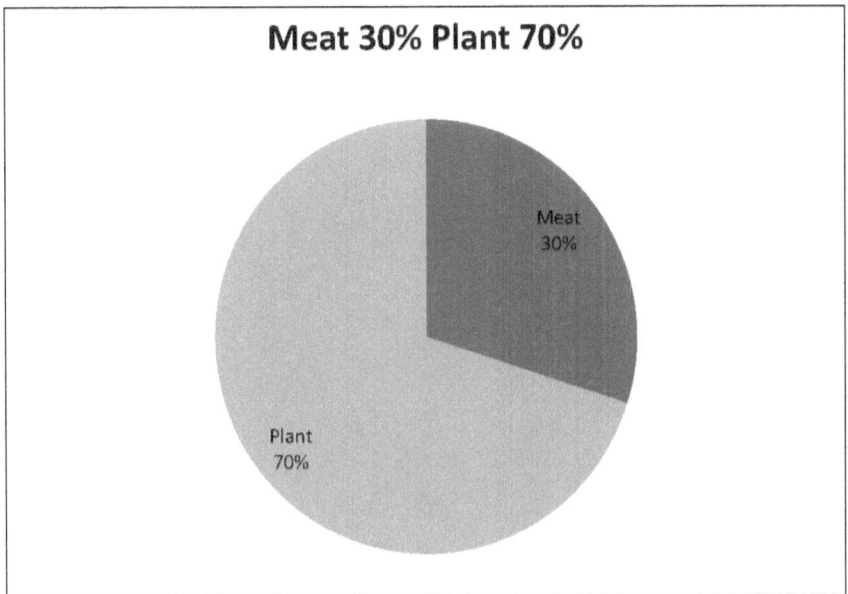

Figure: FNS15

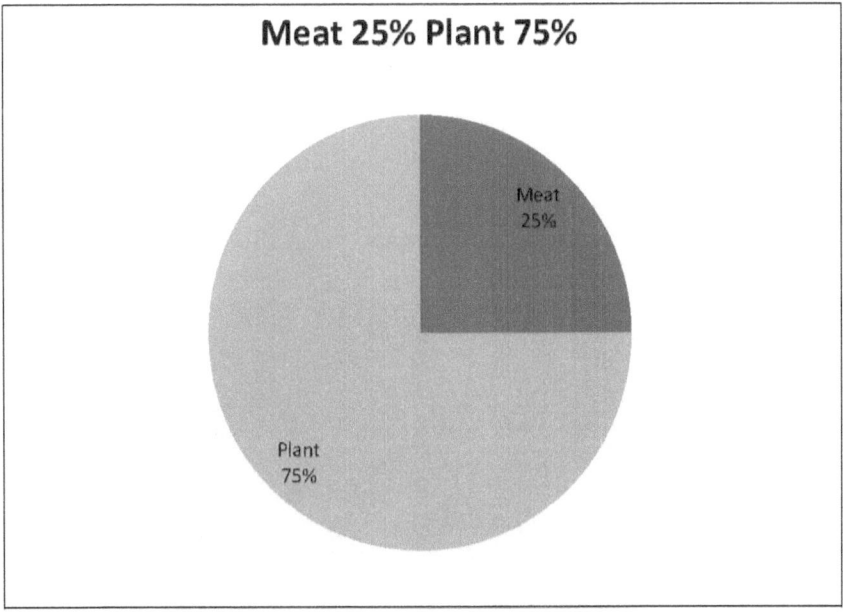

Figure: FNS16

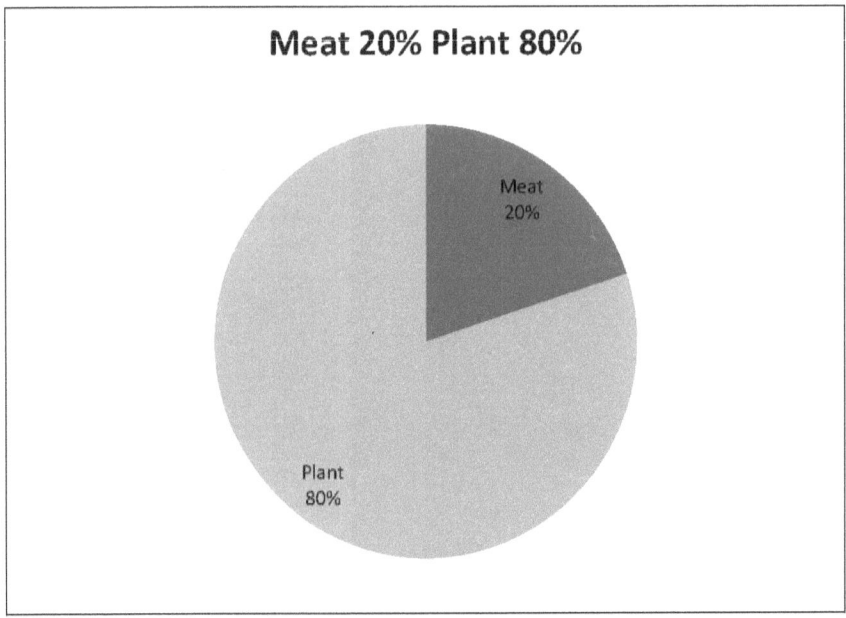

Figure: FNS17

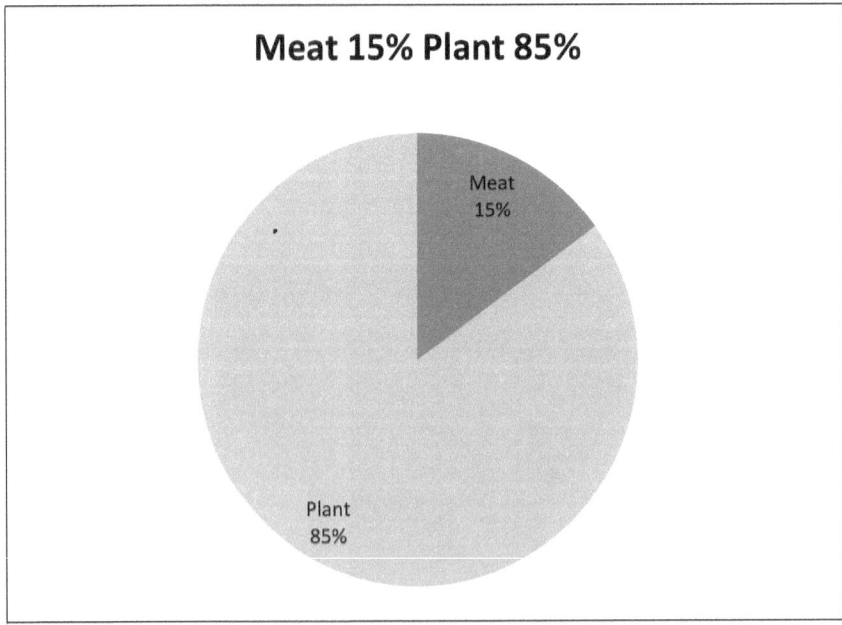

Figure: FNS18

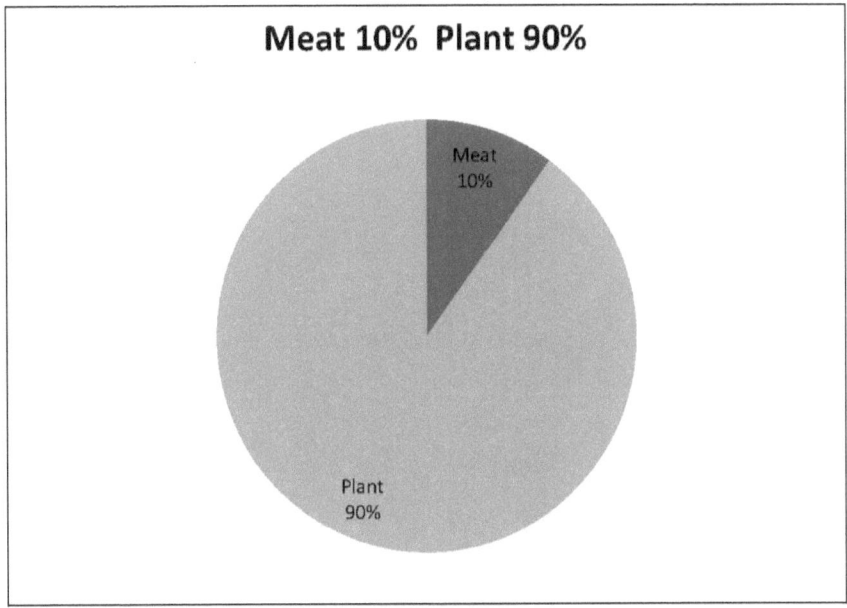

Figure: FNS19

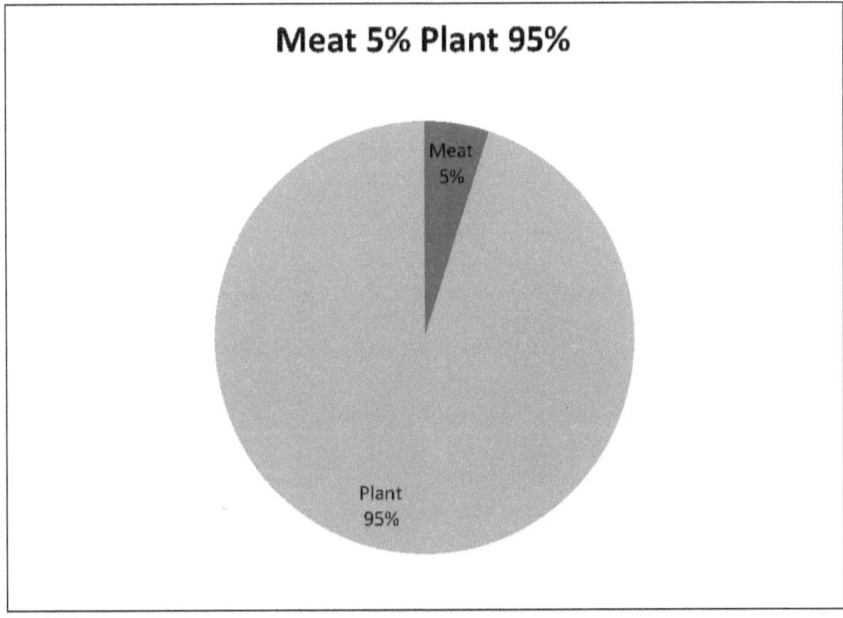

Figure: FNS20

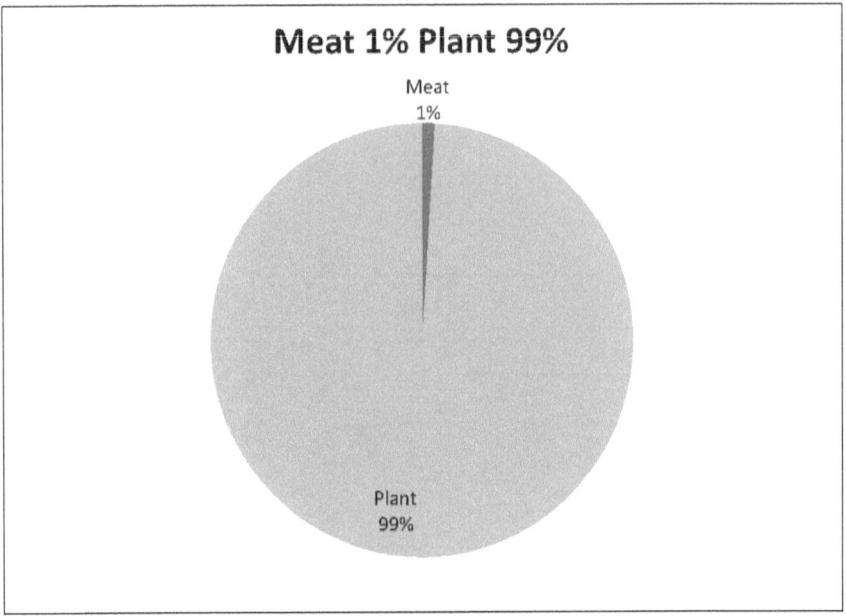

Figure: FNS21

8

Meatarian by Birth: The Meat-Based Diet

Fancy's nutrition spectrum

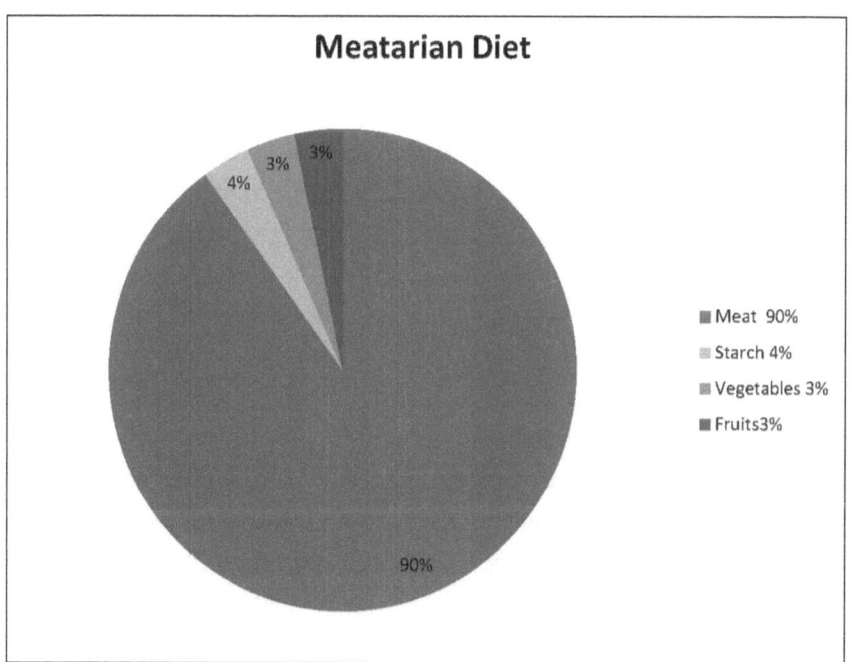

BORN MEATARIAN

Meatarian Diet Basics

The meatarian diet consists of 90 to 99 percent meat. Meat eaters must eat a small portion of any type of vegetable, fruit, and starch each day to be healthy. The preferred drink for this group is milk. A healthy diet for meatarians consists of any variety of meat. This includes poultry, fish, red meats, and so on.

The meatarian diet is the exact opposite of the vegetarian diet.

Natural meatarians who eat a vegetarian diet or a diet made up of the various portions shown in the normal range may develop the following illnesses:

> *Mental illness(violent behavior)* – Some people with mental illness were born meatarian. They must consume a diet of 90 to 99 percent meat and 10 to 1 percent plant food. If they consume more than 10 percent plant food daily, they will become ill. Their sense of reasoning will be impaired.
>
> *Diabetes* – People with diabetes are born meatarians. They must eat a diet of 90 to 99 percent meat and 10 to 1 percent plant food.

The Three-Step Method for Transitioning to a Meatarian Diet

Please note that overcoming diseases using nutrition is not an instantaneous process. It can take from one to five years before you'll see results. Therefore, it is important that, while you are changing your diet you should follow specific guidelines.

The three steps to making this transition are:

1. Eat a meat-only diet for one week.
2. Eat a meatarian diet (95 percent meat, 5 percent plant) for one year.
3. Find the pattern on the nutrition spectrum that works best for you and eat a diet based on that pattern for a lifetime.

A One-Week Meatarian Menu

The following is a suggested menu for one week. No breakfast suggestions are included for day six and seven. People following this diet are encouraged to fast for a period of twelve hours on those days to allow the body to correct itself.

Day 1
   Breakfast
      Eggs
      Bacon
      1/2 slice of bread
      Milk

Lunch
    Chicken
    1 tbsp. Lettuce
    Chocolate Drink

Dinner
    1/4 potato
    1 slice melon
    1 tbsp. collard greens
    Beef
    Milk shake

Day 2
    Breakfast
        Sausage
        1/2 slice bread
        Cherry milk

    Lunch
        Hot dog
        Chocolate milk shake

    Dinner
        Lamb
        1 tbsp. rice
        1slice apple
        1 tbsp. lettuce
        Water

Day 3
    Breakfast
        Ham
        Lettuce
        Goat milk

Lunch
Hamburger patty
Milk

Dinner
Oxtail
1/4 ripe banana
1 tbsp. kale greens
Chocolate milk

Day 4

Breakfast
Broccoli and cheese
Hot cocoa

Lunch
Shrimp
1 tbsps. rice
Milk shake

Dinner
Ribs
1 tbsp. mustard green
1 slice mango
Goat milk

Day 5

Breakfast
Meatballs
Hot Cocoa

Lunch
Salmon
1 tbsp. mustard greens
Water

Dinner
>   Steamed fish
>   1/4 sweet potato
>   1 slice pear
>   Milk

Day 6
>   Breakfast
>   No breakfast

>   Lunch
>   Unsweetened tea
>   Mutton
>   1 tbsp. sweet potatoes
>   Goat milk

>   Dinner
>   Liver and onions
>   1 tbsp. Irish potatoes
>   1 tsp. peanuts
>   Chocolate milk

Day 7
>   Breakfast
>   No breakfast

>   Lunch
>   Ham
>   1/2 slice bread
>   Milk shake

>   Dinner
>   Steak
>   1 tbsp. green beans
>   Milk

9

Vegetarian by Birth: The Plant-Based Diet

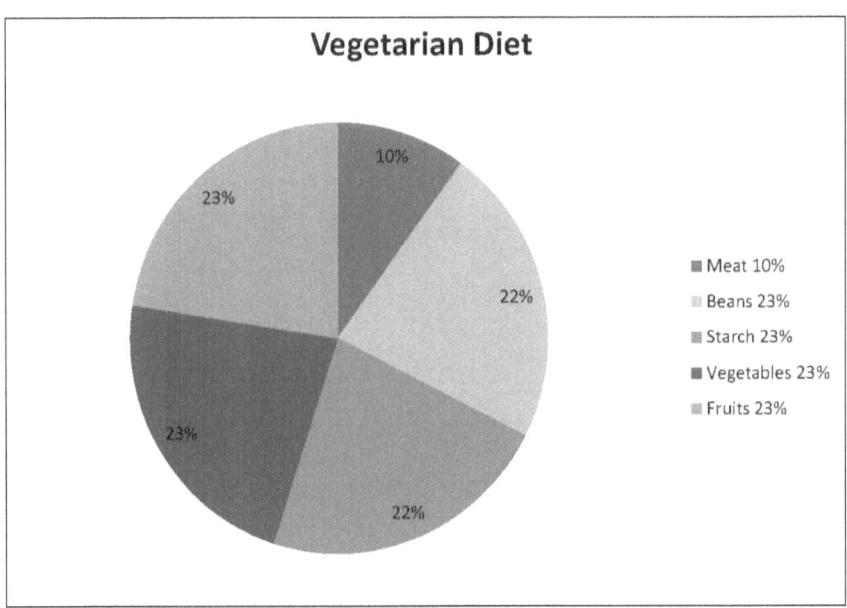

Vegetarian Diet

- Meat 10%
- Beans 23%
- Starch 23%
- Vegetables 23%
- Fruits 23%

BORN VEGETARIAN

Vegetarian Diet Basics

The vegetarian diet consists of 90 percent vegetables and 10 percent meat. Vegetarians must eat meat every day because meat contains vitamin B12, which is not found in plant food.

Vegetarians obtain most of their protein from beans and peas. As often as possible, they should as consume fresh foods from local farmers markets. Vegetarians should drink fruit juices. The vegetarian diet is different from a vegan diet in that a vegan diet contains no animal products whatsoever. For example, a vegan diet excludes eggs and dairy along with meat.

Certain illnesses associated with natural vegetarians include:

Mental Illness (depression) – Some people who are depressed are born vegetarians. They experience depression when they eat too much meat. A depressed person feel like a heavy weight is on him or her. A depressed individual tends reflect on the bad things in life, which makes him or her even more depressed. When people suffering from depression eat a vegetarian diet, the feeling of a heavy weight seems to be lifted off their shoulders. The depressed person should eat lots of fresh fruits from the farmers market. Fruits are full of vitamin C. Consuming lots of fruits is a good method for lifting a depressed mood. I call fresh fruits the happy food. For some people with depression, meat is like wine; if they eat too much meat, they will become mentally impaired.

Stress – Natural vegetarians who eat too much meat can get stressed. For example, a period of intense activity may lead to a period of stress. During severe stress, the person may start hearing voices, make bad choices, feel as though someone is following him or her, or experience insecurity. He or she may try to attack the person they think is responsible for the stress, and his or her sense of reasoning may be off. Severely stressed individuals will very often try to take some drug to reduce these symptoms and end up in a worse place. People who suffer from this kind of stress can eat a vegetarian diet, and all these feelings will go away.

Endometriosis – People who have endometriosis are natural vegetarians. They are born with a weak liver. When they consume too much meat, they have severe pains during their menstrual cycle, and the pain worsens with each menstrual cycle. After pregnancy, the pains increase incrementally until the person experiences severe pains throughout each day. This severe pain occurs mainly on the surface of the left leg, the back of the left hip, and deep in the left waist.

    If people with endometriosis consume a vegetarian diet all the pain in the leg and hip will go away. It seems as if this pain is associated with eating too much meat. If people suffering from this illness avoid oily and fried foods, all the pain in the left waist will be alleviated as well. It seems that this pain is associated with too much oil consumption.

The vegetarian diet should be a lifelong choice for people with endometriosis. When menopause occurs, some people who were on a vegetarian diet to reduce the pain may want to start increasing their intake of meat. However, this is a mistake, as consuming meat will cause the pain symptoms to reoccur.

Slim build (along with inability to gain weight) – People who have slim builds and are unable to gain weight may be vegetarians. It seems that whatever they eat, even if they eat continuously throughout the day and regardless of how large the portions they consume, they are still unable to gain weight. The paradox is the more meat that they eat, the more weight they lose.

Most people think that consuming a vegetarian diet will prevent them from gaining weight. The truth is, if you are a natural vegetarian, eating a vegetarian diet will help you to gain weight.

Backache – Vegetarians who eat too much meat may get backaches. When they stand for a long time, they may experience a pain in their backs. Sometimes the person's back feels as if it's crystallized. When such individuals consume a vegetarian diet, all the backache goes away.

Indigestion – People who are born vegetarians are unable to digest large amount of meat. Therefore, if they consume a large amount of meat, they may have indigestion. Such individuals have to sit in one place for a long time, sometimes up to an hour, to allow the food to digest. Sometimes, the body is unable to process the food even after two to three hours and the person has to take an antacid. And sometimes, even after taking antacid, the person cannot digest the food. The person has to be sick in order to clear the stomach.

Skin disease – If natural vegetarians eat too much meat or milk products, they can get skin rashes, such as eczema or dermatitis. Eating a vegetarian diet will remove these symptoms.

The Three-Step Method for Transitioning to a Vegetarian Diet

Here are three simple steps for changing your diet to a vegetarian only:

1. Eat a vegan diet for one week (plant only)
2. Eat a mostly vegetarian diet (95 percent plant, 5 percent meat) for one year
3. Find the pattern on the nutrition spectrum that is best for you, and eat a diet based on it for a lifetime

A One-Week Vegetarian Menu

The following is a suggested menu for one week. No breakfast suggestions are included for days six and seven. People following this diet are encouraged to fast for a twelve-hour period on these days to allow the body to correct itself.

A mostly vegetarian diet includes beans, which provide proteins; vegetables; starches; fruits; and nuts. In addition, 1 to 5 percent of this diet includes meat.

Day 1
  Breakfast
      Green beans
      1 baked sweet potato
      1 apple
      Orange juice
      Peanuts
      1 egg

  Lunch
      Rice
      Kidney beans
      Collard greens
      Grapes
      Mango juice
      1 tbsp. fish

Dinner
Rice
Navy beans
Mustard greens
1 small chicken leg
2 slices of honeydew melon
Coconut water

Day 2
Breakfast
Sweet peas
Corn on the cob
Kale greens
1 egg
Pistachios
Apple juice

Lunch
Black-eyed peas
Mustard greens
Mashed potatoes
Honeydew melon
Lemonade
1/2 hot dog

Dinner
Lima beans
Brown rice
Broccoli
Strawberries
Fruit punch
2 tbsps. beef

Day 3

    Breakfast

    Pineapple slices

    Black peas

    Cabbage

    Boiled green bananas

    Almonds

    Peach juice

    1/2 sausage

Lunch

    Cherries

    Split peas soup

    Yellow yam

    Plum juice

    2 tbsps. steak

Dinner

    Kiwi

    Shrimp fried rice (1oz. shrimp)

    Grapefruit juice

Day 4

Breakfast

    Black coffee

    Spinach greens

    Snow peas

    Potato

    Pistachio

    Soursop juice

    1 tbsp. tuna

Lunch

    Carrot

    Okra

Eggplant
Dirty rice
Navy beans
Sweetsop juice
2 tbsps. mutton

Dinner
2 tbsps. fish
Pigeon peas
Rice
Sweet potatoes
Collard greens
Tamarind juice

Day 5
Breakfast
Tea
Star apple
Breadfruit
Avocado
Cashew
2 tbsps. scrambled eggs

Lunch
Guinep
Fries
Grape juice
1 tbsp. chicken strip

Dinner
2 tbsps. beef
Broad beans
Yellow rice
Dasheen
Kale greens
Tamarind

Day 6

Breakfast

No breakfast (fasting)

Lunch

Naseberry
Collard greens
Black-eyed peas
Rice and peas
Walnuts
2 tbsps. liver

Dinner

2 tbsps. lamb
Papaya
Rice
Boiled green bananas
Orange juice

Day 7

Breakfast

No breakfast (fasting)

Lunch

Jackfruit
Rice
Butter beans
Orange
Guava juice
2 tbsps. ribs

Dinner

2 tbsps. oxtail
Seasoned rice
Butter beans
Carrot juice

10

Ultimate Nutrition

The ultimate nutrition is when a person is eating the correct combination of meat and plant food. When ultimate nutrition is achieved, you can see the difference by examining various parts of your body. Your heels should be soft. Rough heals are a sign that you need to change the combination of food your consuming. Your skin should be clean and pretty, free from pimples and rashes. Your fingernails should be smooth, and the middle of your hand should soft. Your hair should be healthy and not flaky. The person will be healthy. There will be no backache. Eating the wrong combination of foods can lead to violent outburst of temper.

Nutrition is not magic. It takes a long time to see results. The most important thing is that you can change your nutrition pattern while you are on your medication. The doctor will be able to measure the results and reduce the medication.

How can you find out the correct combination of plant and meat to eat? The best way to find out is to ask your doctor to check your blood sugar level and your protein levels.

Another method of knowing which side of the spectrum you belong to is to determine whether anyone in your family has diabetes. If this is the case, your nutrition will probably be on the meatarian side of the nutrition spectrum. You should be eating more meat than plant food—at least 51 percent of each meal should be meat. If you do not have someone with diabetes in your family, then your ultimate nutrition lies on the vegetarian side of the spectrum. You should eat more plant food than meat, making sure each meal is at least 51 percent plant-based.

If you have someone with diabetes in your family, invest in a blood sugar test kit and test your blood sugar level one hour after a meal. If the test shows that your blood sugar level is too high, increase the amount of meat you eat at the next meal. Take the test again. Start with the plant meat combination FNS10. Decrease the number to FNS9 or lower until the blood sugar level is normal.

In other words, follow this step-by-step process:

A. Determine whether you have a diabetic person in your family.
B. If the answer is yes, eat an FNS10 plant food combination.
C. Take a blood sugar test (ask your doctor to perform the test or use a blood sugar test kit at home)
D. Is your blood sugar normal?
E. If the answer is yes, FNS10 is the correct combination for you.
F. If the answer is no, eat an FNS9 plant food combination.
G. Take another blood sugar test.
H. Is your blood sugar normal?
I. If the answer is yes, FNS10 is the correct combination for you.
J. If the answer is no, eat an FNS8 plan food combination.
K. Take the blood sugar test.
L. Continue decreasing the FNS number until you have found the right combination for you.

If you do not have a person with diabetes in your family, then you should check your protein level. The best method to check your blood protein level is to ask your doctor.

Another way is to check for a protein-related upset stomach following these simple steps:

A. Do you have an upset stomach after eating?
B. If the answer is yes, eat an FNS12 plant food combination.
C. Do you have an upset stomach immediately after eating the FNS12 plant food combination?
D. If the answer is no, this is the correct plant food combination for you.
E. If the answer is yes, eat an FNS13 plant food combination.
F. Do you have an upset stomach immediately after eating the FNS13 plant food combination?

G. If the answer is no, this is the correct plant food combination for you.

H. Continue increasing the FNS number to find the plant-meat combination that works for you (the combination that doesn't leave you with an upset stomach).

11

Dieting

If you decide to go on a diet, it is important to choose the best nutrition pattern. If someone who is born vegetarian selects a diet that contains 90 percent meat and 10 percent plant food, he or she will lose weight but will run the risk of becoming depressed and/or stressed.. If someone is born meatarian and selects a diet that contains 90 percent plant food and 10 percent meat, he or she will lose weight but will run the risk of developing diabetes or mental illness (violent behavior). When dieting, you should choose the diet pattern that is good for you.

One diet, the Daniel Fast, encourages dieters to fast from meats and breads, eating only fruits, vegetables, and lentils. This is a good nutrition choice for people who are born vegetarians, but it is not a good choice for people who are born meatarian.

The best way to diet is:

1) Select the plant/meat pattern that is best for you from Fancy's Nutrition Spectrum.
2) Eat three meals per day.
3) Get at least 20 minutes of sunlight 3 times per day.
4) Exercise outside to ensure that you are getting enough air and enough oxygen.
5) Open all windows to ensure that fresh air from outside is blowing on you twenty-four hours per day.
6) Get enough sleep.

12

Socioeconomic Circumstances and Nutrition

If a person who is born a meatarian eats a vegetarian diet, he or she can develop mental illness; the manifestation of this type of mental illness is that the person may become violent. Also if a person is born a vegetarian and eats a meatarian diet, he or she can develop mental illness; the manifestation of this type of mental illness is depression and, if untreated, may lead to suicide. Violence and suicide are caused by the same thing—a lack of proper nutrition.

In poor communities and poor countries, people tend to eat a mostly plant-based diet, where typically only a small portion of their nutrition comes from meat. This is because meat is very expensive. For a person who is born a vegetarian, eating a mainly plant-based diet will fulfill his or her nutritional needs. However, for a person who is born a meatarian, eating a mainly plant-based diet causes a severe void in terms of meeting his or her nutritional needs and may lead to aggression and violence. Some people eat plant-based diets because of religious beliefs also.

In wealthy countries and communities where there is an abundance of meat, many people tend to eat a meatarian diet. For a person who was born a meatarian, eating a mainly meat-based diet is a very good option. For people who are born vegetarian, this is not a good diet. The severe void in their nutritional needs can lead to depression and suicide. Some persons eat a meatarian diet because of religious reasons.

13

Bible Link

The two types of mental illness identified by Fancy's Nutrition (violent and depression) fits in with the two types of mental illness mentioned in the bible.

In the bible Jesus encountered two types of mentally ill persons. In Mathew 8 vs. 28 (KJV) Jesus encountered two men who were mentally ill. They were violent the bible described them as so fierce that no one could pass that way. This fits the mental illness caused by a person that is born a meatarian and is eating too much plant based food.

In Mathew 17 vs. 15 (KJV) he encountered a man who was mentally ill. This person tried to harm himself by throwing himself in a fire. This fits in with the type of mental illness caused by depression (want to harm oneself) which occurs when a person who is born a vegetarian eats too much meat.

In both circumstances Jesus had compassion on them and healed them.

The plant/meat combination described by Fancy Nutrition Spectrum can be seen in the bible. In John 6 vs. 9 Jesus used five barley loaves and two fishes to feed multitude. Jesus was aware of the nutrition patterns of people and knew that all persons could eat and be full and their nutritional need would be met. The loaves and fishes could feed all nutrition patterns shown on Fancy's Nutrition Spectrum.

14

Fresh Air, Sunlight, and Sleep

Fancy's Air Need Spectrum

Fresh air is important for daily life and for cell health. Fancy's Air Need Spectrum shows the variety of air needed by individuals. The Bible calls it the Breath of Life.

If a fish is taken out of the water, it will start gasping for breath. If it is later returned to water, it will begin breathing again. If some humans are deprived of air, they will become sleepy. If they go outside, they will feel better.

Some humans need lots of air, and some humans can survive on a small amount of air. Those who need more air will faint or become sleepy in enclosed environments with poor ventilation. This is because more air is needed to enable the body to function properly. Some people on the other hand do not require quite so much air for their body to function properly. Poor ventilation can also increase the intensity of diseases.

Fancy's Air Need Spectrum shows the amount of oxygen needed by humans. Some humans need 99 percent fresh air blowing through an open window to get enough oxygen to be healthy. This is equivalent to being outside. How can this be achieved in a closed environment? Ensure that your environment has lots of windows and doors and that the windows and doors are open. This will ensure that air is flowing through the room you are in at all times. There must be open windows and doors on all sides of the building to enable movement of air throughout the building.

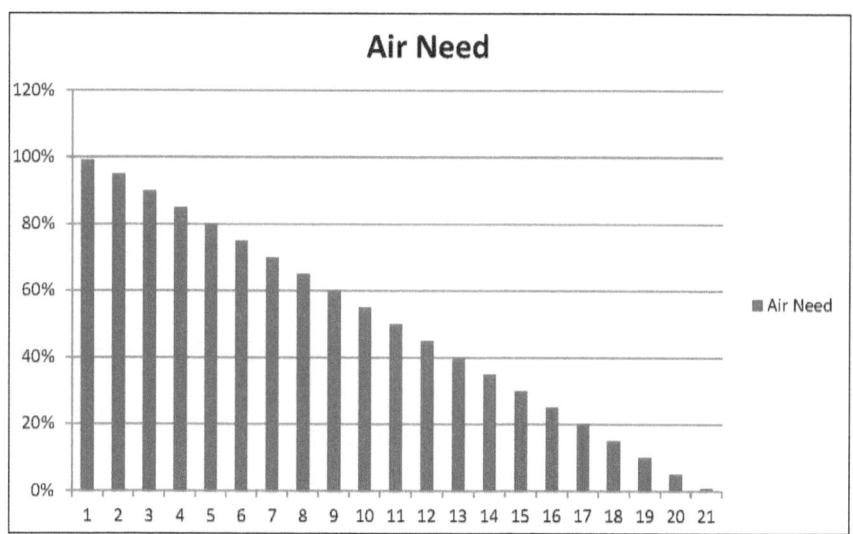

Fancy's Air Need Spectrum

Air moves in a straight line or in a circular pattern, for example, in a hurricane. People need to be in an environment where air is flowing all the time. Thus, for air to circulate properly in an enclosed environment, it must flow in a straight line or in a circular pattern. Air does not circulate properly in buildings with passages that lead to a dead end. Air circulates poorly in a large room unless the windows and doors are opened.

Open your windows and let in the breath of life.

Fancy's Sun Need Spectrum

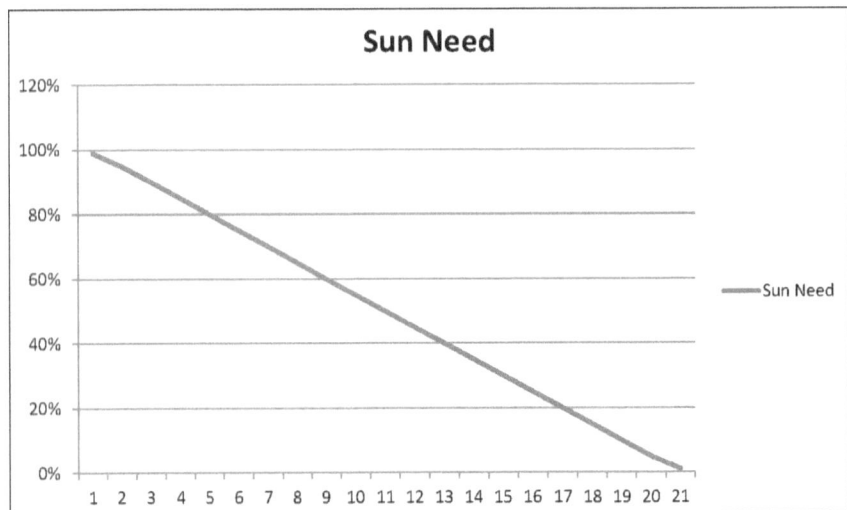

Fancy's Sun Need Spectrum

Fancy's Sun Need Spectrum shows people's various needs for sunlight.

Our bodies need sunlight. Sunlight is necessary for several body functions, including the synthesis of vitamin D. Some people need to be in the sunlight more than others.

Many individuals may find themselves working or living in an environment where a sufficient amount of air and sunlight isn't available. It is important for these individuals to go outside at least three times per day for twenty minutes in order to get enough fresh air and sunlight.

The strongest plants are in the forest, not in the office. This is because the plants in the forest get 100 percent fresh air and sunlight and, so, grow up to be strong and healthy. The plants in the office are usually weak.

Sleep

People with endometriosis need to get a lot of sleep, as one of the problems that result from endometriosis is stress. For people who suffer from stress, proper nutrition, adequate airflow (open windows), and adequate sleep are particularly important.

Setting a few sleep parameters can help ensure these individuals get adequate sleep. First, plan enough time for sleep—plan to sleep for at least nine hours per day. Second, find a bedtime that works best for you (the time that allows you to get eight hours of uninterrupted sleep). It is important to go to sleep at the same time every day. One thing that can disturb sleep is the change that occurs with daylight saving time. To get around this, you will have to change your bedtime during daylight saving time. For example, if you regularly sleep between 8:00 p.m. and 5:00 a.m., then during daylight saving time, you will have to sleep between 9:00 p.m. and 6:00 a.m. This will ensure that you are sleeping during the same period each day. Finally, some foods may cause you to be unable to sleep. It is important to discover what these foods are and eliminate them from your diet or avoid eating them close to bedtime.

Conclusion

Endometriosis is a painful disease. The severe pains associated with this illness occur when a woman has her monthly cycle. Eating a mostly vegetarian diet (one that includes about one tablespoon of any type of meat per meal) and reducing the amount of oil in your diet can reduce these pains. Getting lots of fresh air and eight hours of sleep also help.

During the process of finding the solution for endometriosis, I discovered that a vegetarian diet can also alleviate stress and depression. I learned, too, that human nutrition lies on a spectrum, which I have diagrammed in a model I call Fancy's Nutrition Spectrum. This model shows that we are each born with a body chemistry that determines how we should eat to ensure we are receiving the ultimate nutrition—for each of us, that perfect diet lies somewhere along a spectrum, in terms of a combination of plant food and meat. It is important to know which diet is best for you, just like it is important to know your dress size or shoes size. On one end of the spectrum is the vegetarian diet, where a person eats a primarily plant-based diet, along with a tablespoonful of any type of meat per meal. The meatarian diet, on the other end of the spectrum, is the exact opposite of the vegetarian diet. A meatarian diet consists primarily of meat, along with a tablespoonful of plant food per meal.

Once you have found the plant-meat combination on Fancy's Nutrition Spectrum that works for you, it will be your diet for your entire life. Of course, unusual circumstances may occur that may cause slight variations. Air supply, sunlight, and sleep are also important for good health. Some people need more oxygen than others do. To be healthy, humans must ensure they are eating the proper combination of meat and plant food and that they have sufficient oxygen and sunlight and sleep.

When I've explained the theory of Fancy's Nutrition Spectrum, I've received an array of feedback:

1) Some people laugh at the theory.

2) Some people say they love meat too much to reduce the amount they are eating.
3) Some people say that they will only do what their doctors say.
4) Some people with mental illness (violent behavior)) have started eating more meat and have not had any more psychotic episodes.
5) Some people have eaten less meat and have reduced indigestion and pains from endometriosis.

What will your reaction be?

References

Eating with the Seasons by Paula Bartimeus
Feed Your Body Right by Lendon H. Smith, MD
Real Food for Healthy Kids by Tanya Wenman Steel

www.ingramcontent.com/pod-product-compliance
Lightning Source LLC
Chambersburg PA
CBHW030519290526
45786CB00004B/1534